Herbal Healing for Men

Use Herbs to Rejuvenate Your Body, Combat Exhaustion, and Increase Libido

By

Amanda Goldsmith

Herbal Healing for Men

Copyright © 2019

All rights reserved. This book or any portion thereof may not be reproduced or used in any manner whatsoever without the express written permission of the publisher except for the use of brief quotations in a book review.

ISBN: 9781698907437

Warning and Disclaimer

Every effort has been made to make this book as accurate as possible. However, no warranty or fitness is implied. The information provided is on an "as-is" basis. The author and the publisher shall have no liability or responsibility to any person or entity with respect to any loss or damages that arise from the information in this book.

MEDICAL DISCLAIMER: All information, content, and material of this book is for informational purposes only and are not intended to serve as a substitute for the consultation, diagnosis, and/or medical treatment of a qualified physician or healthcare provider.

Publisher contact

Skinny Bottle Publishing

books@skinnybottle.com

**SKINNY
BOTTLE**

Introduction

The year that Viagra was introduced in the market was a revelation. Millions of prescriptions were written for sexual maladies laying bare many health issues plaguing modern men. At large are serious diseases like cardiac arrest, hypertension, diabetes, prostate issues, infertility, and impotence. It's unfortunate but fewer men are visiting the doctor for screenings. Men were mostly ignoring life-threatening symptoms. Men were more inclined to practice self-medication, and appeared reluctant to exercise, diet and follow good healthcare practices. Obviously, the American male was not in the pink of health, and treatment got postponed till symptoms became too chronic to ignore.

The root cause of male suffering

The problem with men is their reluctance to face personal health issues and the ego that avoids professional counseling. Men are generally less inclined to discuss their sexual issues fearing a backlash from near and dear ones. There are recorded instances of sportsmen playing on regardless of severe physical pain. Ultimately, these men ended up with chronic health issues that nipped budding careers. Perhaps it's because men are physically and emotionally conditioned to appear strong and to not cry over disabilities no matter how serious they may be. To seek professional counseling was to appear weak and infirm or worse to be unmanly. This attitude cocoons men from family and friends and their larger social circle. In this manner, men's health issues and healthcare took a backseat in the hurry burry of routine life.

Men and the art of herbal healing

The majority of men turn to the western system of Allopathic medicine. Allopathic doctors specializing in various branches of healthcare use powerful drugs to relieve pain, remove physical distress, mend broken bones, and cure potent diseases. Modern medicine is symptomatic in its treatment, with little or no emphasis on preventive healthcare. There is little or no counseling related to self-help. Doctors usually don't explain how men could follow preventive healthcare and how they could boost the body's self-curative mechanisms. In short, modern western medicine, as it is practiced today, doesn't take a holistic view of men's problems. Short of prescribing powerful medication, the medical system doesn't consider a man's mental and emotional wellbeing.

To state the obvious, we aren't discrediting the huge progress achieved by modern medicine. Scientific and institutional research in Allopathic fields has significantly reduced the outbreak of serious disease. Life-threatening diseases are under control. Chronic ailments are being treated, and pain is more bearable. The benefits of modern medicine have impacted the lives of millions of people.

Herbal medicine breaks new ground by viewing a man holistically (body, mind, and spirit). Herbalists teach a man to take care of himself, promoting his wellbeing in a holistic way. Herbal science teaches us that man has closely bonded with nature, and the human body has evolved best by closely associating with plants, flowers, fruits, and herbs. The herbalist will tell you that you can draw deep from the curative power of sunshine, oxygen and the food that nature has provided in abundance as we have been accustomed to do for uncounted centuries.

It is a myth that herbal healing for men is completely divorced from modern medicine. The truth is that both systems complement each other remarkably. It is wrong to ignore one system and to promote the other. What men need to do is to accept the best that each system has to offer. Men must harness natural curative powers that heal the body. Herbal healing lowers drug dependence without side effects.

Happily, men today are realizing the potential of herbal medicine and yoga, two potent tools for healing mind, body, and soul. It also helps that a great deal of research is revealing the healing powers of common herbs. It is heartening that American men are turning to holistic herbal healing in a big way to complement what modern medicine offers.

Empowering men's health through herbal remedies

The sheer variety of herbal medication

Herbs lose their mystery once you create the perfect remedy with your own hands. It doesn't matter if you can't cook; what's more important is that you know what you are dealing with. All you need to do is to follow the simple recipes that we've put together in this book. Some of the biggest names and businesses in herbal medication belong to men (and women of course) who learned the art of herbal healing without basic cooking skills.

The advantage of herbal medicine is that you can apply the potion in many forms – as teas that soothe, tinctures that awaken, and as pills that are easy to swallow. Creativity is at its best when you experiment with syrupy sweet elixirs, delicious jam or jelly-like potions, and powdery substances that can be sweetened with honey. No other medicine comes in such attractive packages.

Leave aside the herbal medicine that you take orally; there are hundreds of poultices, compresses, and oils that apply the healing touch. With herbs, you get a free hand to tackle any health issue. Whether it's sore muscles or sprains, or bruises and cuts, herbal healing is safe, effective, and long-lasting.

Studying and selecting the right herbs

It is not enough to source an herb from the local market. You need to study its potency and quality. You can make a beginning by asking the grower whether the plant was grown in an eco-friendly way without GM inputs, fertilizers, and pesticides. An herb that is grown on poor quality soil will be less effective. Ask about the herb's harvesting and drying methods to assess whether the product is ecologically safe.

It is possible to study the freshness of an herb using all the senses as you would when buying vegetables in an open market. An herb should be visually attractive, retaining all if not most of its color and vibrancy. Study the herb in its natural environment and assess whether the dried version retains its original color. The same applies to blossoms, fruits, leaves, stems, and roots.

What makes the herb unique is its distinctive smell. Not all herbs are sweet-smelling. Some are potent and pungent. It should smell as fresh as the day it was harvested and dried. Some smells like that of valerian repel, while peppermint will smell refreshing.

Tasting gives you direct feedback on the herb's freshness and potency. Fresh herbs will excite the taste buds with extreme sweetness or pungency. The stronger the effect on the tongue, the fresher will be the herb. The best way to learn is to see, smell, and taste herbs in their natural surroundings.

Preserving herbs in dried form

The best way to preserve herbs is to store them in airtight containers in dark and cool places; you need to protect them from pests, air, light, heat, and moisture. If you follow these basic precautions, you'll see your herbal farm giving you years' worth of unending supplies.

Just how much of an herb is safe to consume?

Modern medicine delivers ingredients in precise doses, but the same isn't true of herbs. Herbal healing depends a lot on your personal knowledge and experience in handling ingredients in the correct way. Too small a dosage can be ineffective, whereas too big a dose could be disastrous. The dosages that we mention in this book are based on years of experience. The herbalist prepares remedies that'll be unique to you and your height, weight and physical condition. He will carefully note your past history of ailments or chronic conditions. It's important to be aware of allergies that heighten your sensitivity to certain herbs.

Being mindful of the effects of herbal healing

For safety, only the finest herbs that have a known history of benefits (minus side effects) have been mentioned in this book. Toxic herbs or herbs that produce excessive tissue reactions have been completely avoided as these ingredients can be consumed only under professional supervision. Dry eyes, sore skin that breaks into rashes, an upset tummy or a feeling of dehydration are symptoms that warn you to discontinue herbal treatment.

Trusted remedies in herbal healing for men

Herbal tea extracts

Preparing an herbal concoction or tea is perhaps the simplest way of extracting the benefits. It doesn't involve any specialized knowledge or skill. Even a novice can do it without breaking a sweat.

Boiling an herb is not the best method of extraction. Essential oils and vital ingredients tend to break down at high temperatures. The fleshy parts of herbs such as leaves and flowers are packed with oils that are best extracted through infusion. In this technique we gently pour hot (not boiling) water over the herb, allowing the mixture to steep in the warmth for an hour. If you increase the quantity of the herb and prolong the infusion time, you end up with a more potent brew. The most effective treatments require a strongly brewed tea. Usually, the right quantity will be a cup of water for every spoonful of herb.

The harder parts of the herb such as its bark, roots, and stems need a stronger extraction method called decoction. Using the same measure as in the infusion method, heat a mixture of cold water and herbs to simmering point. Prolong simmering for about 45 minutes over a low flame. The mixture is allowed to cool overnight. The brewed tea is then consumed after straining the herb. Whether you are steeping through the infusion method or brewing using the decoction technique, a heat exposure of 30 to 45 minutes is essential to create a stronger brew. Seal the tea in airtight jars to prevent essential nutrients from escaping via steam.

Herbal extracts in pill and capsule form

If you find it difficult to drink brews that are strongly flavored, an easy way out is to consume herbal extracts as pills. Do a quality check by opening the capsule to test the powder's texture, smell, and taste. Ensure that the capsule is of vegetable origin because the gelatin made from animal products may be harder to digest. You'll find they don't dissolve as easily as the vegetable counterpart. Last but not the least; ensure that the company manufacturing the pills follows high-quality standards.

Herbal pastes

If you can't access high-quality capsules, the better alternative is to make a fine paste of powdered herbs. A delightful pasty consistency can be achieved by mixing the powdered herbs with maple syrup, and honey and in adding nutmeg and cinnamon or cardamom. Prepared this way, the herbal paste can be stored in airtight containers for longer periods. A spoonful of the paste can be consumed as a tea after adding to hot water or used as a spread over toast and crackers.

Whole plant herbal extraction

Though a lot of research is in advanced stages, we're still unsure which active ingredient is performing the healing role. We also don't know whether it is one single ingredient or a combination of ingredients that is doing the healing. For this reason, it would be great if the entire plant is used in the extraction technique instead of focusing only on individual parts. This ensures that the herbal extract contains all active ingredients in the right potency and combination that is ready for healing.

Maximizing potency of herbs through tinctures

Decoctions and infusions are great where a fresh herbal batch can be quickly processed for instant use. Pills containing powdered herbs are useful when it's necessary to preserve the herbal product over a longer period. The tincture method is best when you want to achieve stronger herbal potency. A few drops of the concentrated herbal extract can be mixed with warm water, teas or fruit and vegetable juices throughout the day. For preparing a tincture, you need a strong extractant. The most powerful extractant is alcohol used in minute quantities. If you're not Ok with alcohol, vegetable-based glycerin or apple cider vinegar are low potency extractants. Tinctures are marvelous because they enjoy the longest shelf life, but you need to follow the dosage instructions carefully.

Tinctures can be easily prepared using any of the following ways:

Blending: Both fresh and dried parts of the herbal plant are shredded minutely, mixed with the chosen extractant and blended using a mixer grinder.

Mixing: in this technique, take the shredded herbs in a small-sized jar and let the chosen extractant cover the mixture by around three inches. Liquors like brandy and vodka make excellent extractants. Glycerin of vegetable origin can also be used in 50:50 ratios with water. Another method is to employ apple cider vinegar that can be warmed and added to the herbal mixture. Cover the jar tightly for maximizing herbal potency.

Slow soaking: The herbal plant is shredded and soaked in the extractant in a jar stored in warm surroundings. Soaking is permitted for up to six weeks to achieve the highest potency. The jar must be shaken occasionally to ensure that the herbs don't settle at the bottom.

Precautions to be taken

Ensure to label the jars, naming the contents and entering the date when soaking began. This gives you an idea of how long the herbs have been soaked. Use a coarse muslin cloth to strain the mixture and remove the solid particles when soaking is over. Don't forget to label the tincture so you are aware of what you're consuming.

Preparing herbal oils and salves

Herbal oils that are commercially prepared are nothing but herbs mixed in an oily medium such as olive oil. The problem is that you won't know how concentrated the herb is. The safer method is to make your own herbal oil using fresh herbs. Freshly dried herbs with the lowest water content make the best oils and salves. If you are harvesting fresh plant parts, it's best that you lay them out on a coarse towel out in the shade. Simply allow the herbs to dry out completely over a couple of hours. Lower water content paves the way for the efficient extraction of herbal ingredients. This is the best method for preparing a potent herbal oil infusion.

Infusing herbs in oil using a double boiler

The easier way of infusing herbal oils is to use a medium-sized double boiler with one pot positioned over the other. This way, you can boil water in the lower pot, keeping herbs in the upper pot soaked in oil. It's better not to expose the herb and oil mixture to your burner. Steam heating through the double boiler method prevents the oil from burning and herbs from frying.

Immerse the herbs in the upper pot in an inch or two of olive oil. Take a reasonable quantity of water in the lower pot, allowing the water to simmer after reaching the boiling point. Allow the herbs to soak in oil for an hour. The gentle and prolonged simmering creates a concentrated infusion, making the herbal oils darker, besides giving off a strong scent.

After infusing, allow the herbal oil to cool and use a fine muslin cloth to strain the solid particles. You may discard the used herbs and store the freshly prepared oil in an airtight container which should be properly labeled.

Using solar power to infuse herbal oils

This is the technique favored by our ancestors for making potent herbal infusions. You'll see most Mediterranean countries using this method. Sandboxes are prepared for storing numerous jars containing the herb and oil mixtures. Ensure that the oil covers the herbal plant by around two to three inches, and then store the closed jars in the sandboxes over a prolonged period. The natural heat generated by the sun efficiently infuses the primary herbal ingredients into the oil. If you want, you can discard the used herbs and add fresh herbs after a decent interval. You end up with doubly potent herbal oil with greater medicinal value.

Herbal oils infused in the solar way seem to last much longer than ordinary infusions and do not turn rancid quickly.

Precautions to be taken

It is possible that a moist climate may induce droplets of water to condense inside the closed jar. One way of reducing moisture is to wrap the mouth of the jar with cheesecloth before tightening the cap.

Storage becomes an issue because herbal oils turn rancid and become unusable as the infusion ages. The best way out is to use coconut oil or olive oil which are stable extractants and to store jars in darker, cooler places away from direct sunlight and in doubly sealed containers.

Preparing herbal ointments or salves

If you've had your fill of tinctures, the next big step is to move on to herbal ointments that have a variety of uses. Salves or ointments as they are mostly called are concentrated herbal preparations thickened with oil and beeswax.

After infusing and straining the herbal oil, take one cup of herbal oil and mix it with a quarter cup of grated beeswax. Again, using a fresh pot, gently warm (don't boil) the mixture till you see the beeswax melting and becoming thicker. There's a simple way of judging the quality of either oil or beeswax. Scoop a tablespoon of the ointment and place it in the freezer for a couple of minutes. Then rub the ointment between your fingers. If the salve is too hard, this indicates lower oil content which can be remedied by adding more oil. If the ointment is too soft, you need more beeswax. Add the ingredients in small samples, alternately warming and cooling the mixture till you get the right thickness.

Precautions to be taken

As you'll be handling very hot mixtures, take care to prevent scalding. Store only in airtight and sterilized bottles stored in cool and dark cupboards to prolong the life of the medication. Remember that exposure to air and sunlight spoil ointments, darkening and diminishing their effectiveness.

The simplicity of preparing a refreshing herbal bath

Taking a shower is not half as refreshing as the traditional tub bath. There's something relaxing and rejuvenating about a tubful of warm water, especially if you add some herbal magic to liven up things. Cool water has a stimulating effect that freshens up the body for a stressful day. Warm water has a relaxing effect loosening knots and muscle cramps to ease the strain of a hard day.

It's easy to create an herbal bath, and all you have to do is to tie up a bunch of fresh or dried herbs into a silk or nylon sock and hang it over the tub nozzle right under a slow stream of warm water. Later as the tub fills the same sock can be unhooked and floated in the water, its herbal oils and active ingredients soaking the water completely. Another method is to place the herbal concoction in a tea strainer or closed tea ball with a metal chain fastening it to the nozzle of the tub, and exposing the contents to a steady stream of warm water.

Applying herbs externally to the body

The herbal compress is designed for stimulating and medicating the body from the outside. In this process, strong tea of an herbal mix is either cold-pressed or hot-pressed to the surface of the skin to get the proper result. The heated herb draws out impurities in the skin and improves blood circulation, especially in areas that are sore and cramped. The compress can be very useful in soothing sunburns, relieving cramps, healing bruises, and reducing inflammation.

The best method of preparing a hot compress is to use roughly thrice the amount of herbs that you would use in a tea. You can tie up the herbs in a soft muslin cloth bag sealed at one end. The muslin bag is then heated in the upper pot of a double potboiler. A cold compress can be easily prepared by repeating the process and by cooling the muslin bag in a fridge for a couple of minutes.

You can also use a hot water bottle or a pan of iced water to alternatively heat or cool the herbal bag. The compress is then placed gently over the affected part until the heat or cold dissipates. The process can be repeated throughout the day and can be used to complement the herbal medication or tea that you consume orally.

Direct application of herbs or pastes over the skin

Herbs can also be applied fresh, grated, mashed or mixed with fresh clay over the skin in affected parts of the body. Such a process would be called a poultice. This is very effective when you're treating insect bites, rashes, boils, and pimples as well as swollen glands. Body parts with internal tumors and swellings respond well to this treatment. The active ingredients in the herbal mix penetrate deeply via skin pores. To boost the healing process, boil the herbs into a mushy pulp making it easier to apply externally. To prevent the herbal mix from leaking away at the sides, cover the poultice with a moist cloth. Cotton materials and soft towels are best. After soaking the skin over a short period, replace the poultice and repeat. A hot water bottle or a bag of ice cubes works just as well to heat or cool the poultice.

Herbal healing in men: the art of rejuvenating the body

Herbal mixes prepared on the lines of well-established formulae are truly great. They are health-enhancing tonics that are a must-have for men looking to soothe tired bodies and exhausted spirits.

Ginger and turmeric enhanced herbs coated with dark chocolate

The attractiveness of herbal medication lies in the complete freedom one enjoys in enhancing or reducing its sugar content. Spicing up an herbal mix with turmeric adds power to its anti-inflammatory effect. Turmeric aids neuro-muscular coordination, mental health, bone rejuvenation, and heart health besides strengthening the body's immune system enabling it to fight serious diseases and infection. For maximizing the health benefits create a fresh batch of turmeric that has been thoroughly dried and powdered. Ginger is an excellent digestive and goes a long way in checking gastro-intestinal disease and GERD. You can also add powerful herbs such as ashwagandha that tackle sexual issues and promote vitality.

Place a double potboiler over a burner boiling sufficient water in the lower pan. Take three-quarters of a teacup of coconut oil in the upper pan to which you add twice the measure of shredded dark chocolate. Melt the chocolate over low heat, stirring the upper pan constantly, till you achieve a pasty semiliquid (pourable) texture. Remove the upper pan and add optional ingredients such as turmeric powder (half cup), grated ginger (quarter cup), crushed walnuts (one cup), freshly crushed black pepper (one spoon), vanilla extract(one spoon), and half a spoon of unrefined sea salt. You can also add dried fruits such as raisins for a full-bodied flavor and texture. Pour the semiliquid mixture into a candy mold and leave it to cool and solidify. The dried candy lasts longer if you store it in an airtight container in the fridge. Consume at least one or two candy bits on a daily basis.

Herbal energy balls and bars

Medicated herbal candies are great for sugar coating healing actions but the fun doesn't end there. You can also prepare delightful energy snacks using herbs. An herbal energy ball can deliver a three-fold benefit by stimulating your endocrine glands, replace lost vitamins and nutrients, besides providing a much-needed energy boost that'll carry you through a busy day.

Preparation

Prepare a smooth paste mixing tahini (two cups with the oil skimmed off), nut butter (two cups of almonds, peanuts or cashew nuts) and honey (I to 2 cups according to taste). Take a bowl and mix the paste and herbs well. Add finely grated walnuts or almond (or both) to the herbal mixture, introducing a cup of grated coconut and two cups of chocolate chips. Now add an ounce each of maca, ashwagandha, eleuthero, and Rhodiola powders. At this stage, you can optional ingredients such as dried cranberries or raisins flavored with goji berries. Unsweetened cocoa powder or melted chocolate will thicken the herbal mixture. Using hands mix all the ingredients thoroughly, creating a thickened dough. Now roll up the dough into medium-sized balls and you're ready to impart a light coating. Simply roll the balls in a liquid mix of cocoa powder or a tray of melted chocolate and finish off with a sprinkling of lightly toasted and grated coconut. You can store the energy balls in an airtight container using parchment paper to separate the balls. Two balls daily separated by a 12-hour timeframe will give you all the energy you need to speed up a busy day.

Adding pep to herbal energy balls

Adding an ounce each of guarana and kola nut powders is a great way to pep up an energy ball. The high caffeine content (higher than coffee) of guarana is a great way to get an instant mood boost and to enhance athletic prowess.

Energy balls are a great way of enhancing moods and staying fit and active. These simple recipes can be experimented with using passion inducing Chambord and aphrodisiac herbs such as ginseng, ginger, and damiana. The only word of caution is that men prone to hypertension, heart disease, and diabetes should go easy on energy balls. Keep track of basic health parameters – sugar, heartbeat, blood pressure – when you are consuming energy balls to ensure they are safe for you.

The curative and rejuvenating powers of maca

If you're searching for an herb that strengthens the immune system and injects stamina and vitality to your sex life, that search ends with maca. Its tasty butterscotch like flavor makes maca quite addictive.

Prepare a smooth and creamy paste of half a cup of nut butter and a quarter cup of honey, stirring in half a cup of maca powder. Cocoa powder is an excellent ingredient that thickens the dough considerably. Scoop the dough into medium-sized balls that can be stored in the fridge wrapped in parchment paper and stored in airtight containers. For a nutty chocolaty flavor dip the balls in cocoa paste or melted chocolate before drying storing. Two balls daily will add spice to the most ordinary day and your partner won't complain if you become over-attentive.

The versatility of herbal powders

Man's search for the instant 'fix' ends with herbal powders that can be consumed in a variety of ways. The beauty of herbal powders is that they can be added to all kinds of fruit and vegetable juices, soups and smoothies. The simplest recipe would be steeping herbal powders in hot water. To prepare a power-packed herbal powder, mix ashwagandha, eleuthero, maca, and yam powders, taking mot more than an ounce of each ingredient. A strong tea made of this herbal mix (spoon or two daily) rejuvenates reproductive functioning, besides reducing stress and boosting the immune system. The tea makes for a strong drink that boosts health and wellbeing. Licorice powder is an excellent addition if you are not on blood pressure or heart meds.

The all-powerful health-restoring herbal shake

Rhodiola, kava, and ashwagandha are herbal ingredients that give a terrific pep up keeping you in high spirits throughout a busy day. Mix almond milk, maca, eleuthero, and Rhodiola powders along with a ripe banana, along with a handful of blueberries and raw pumpkin seeds in a mixer, adding a healthy dose of maple syrup and a spoon of vanilla extract. The resulting blend is a great nourished and organ cleanser.

High energy, high protein foods that enhance male power

•	Tomatoes lightly sautéed in olive oil give you a healthy dose of lycopene that stimulates the prostate gland and prevents cancer.

•	Cauliflower, cabbage, and broccoli promote bladder health and prevent the onset of cancer in the male reproductive system.

•	Green leafy veggies with loads of vitamins and antioxidants do a great job in protecting the body against cancers, and inflammation. They enhance immune function and aid digestion.

•	Organically grown fruits are a treasure chest of vitamins, minerals, and fiber. A daily dose of fresh-cut or juiced fruit is an excellent detoxifier and liver protector.

•	Sesame seeds along with tahini offer loads of calcium and healthy fats that protect the nervous system and strengthen bones.

•	Pumpkin seeds are an excellent source of zinc, an essential ingredient boosting male sexual health.

• Buttermilk and yogurt abundant in probiotic cultures replenish healthy bacteria that reside in the gut and aid digestion.

• Fish are an abundant source of heart-healthy omega-6 fatty oils and protein. Regular consumption of fish promotes heart health, boosts brainpower, and counters nervous disorders and depression.

• Oysters, high in zinc content are a powerful aphrodisiac boosting reproductive health. Just three helpings of oysters will keep you sexually active and happy.

The all-purpose herbal elixir of life

Mix together one measure each of Muira Puama and sarsaparilla root, one-fourth teaspoon of cinnamon chips, a quarter measure of dried ginger powder, three cardamom pods, a cup of any liquor (vodka, brandy or dark rum), and any fruit concentrate to your liking. Follow our recipe for creating a strong tincture and then add black cherry concentrate. Your all-purpose health rejuvenating elixir is now ready for consumption. Add a spoon or two of the elixir to water, smoothies or fruit juice and let the herbs do their magic. A note of caution is to use fruit concentrates (not juices) to prevent the elixir from fermenting. Where possible, use fresh cut herbs that don't leave a residue like powders. The elixir is exquisite, leaving a fruity aftertaste, and men can be excused for labeling it as the elixir of the Gods.

The love potion that will steam up sensuous nights

You might find it hard to believe but a simple cup of dried damiana is all that is essentially required to fire up your spirits and sexual energy. So, before your date turns up for the momentous occasion use this potent potion to perk up the night. Believe us, your partner may find it equally hard to say no to this recipe. Take a cupful of dried damiana leaves and let then stew in two cups of dark brandy in a covered glass jar for a period not less than five days. Now sieve the soaked damiana leaves and transfer to another clean jar filled with one and a half cups of clear mineral water. Allow the liquor-soaked damiana leaves to rest for three days in the covered jar. Now warm the strained damiana infused water over very low heat stirring in a cup of honey; once the mixture is cool add the earlier infused brandy, and a spoon each of vanilla and rose extract. Store the herbal infusion in a tightly sealed jar for a month, allowing the brew to mellow gently. Reserve the potent aphrodisiac for that all-important drink serving it to your partner as well and enjoy the soothing sensuousness of the drink as the night sets in. Adding half a cup of melted chocolate, almonds or rose water heightens the potency making it a treat for those with a sweet tooth.

The herbal wine that's a treat for all occasions

Red and white wines make delightful combinations with a playful infusion of choicest herbs. This recipe enhances sexual energy and keeps you stress-free and smarter when happy hour approaches. Mix a quarter cup of dried damiana, three-quarters of a cup full of horny goat weed (or Rhodiola if you wish), three-quarters of a cup of wholegrain oats, adding one whole vanilla bean and two cardamom pods. Use a clean glass jar covering the herbal mixture with three inches of wine (more if necessary as the herbs swell). Allow the mixture to infuse the wine for up to three weeks. Then strain away from the herbs and repackage the wine in a new bottle ready for instant use. You can small amounts of ginger, cinnamon, cloves, and black pepper to make the wine spicier.

The cider stimulant

Ever experienced a kind of sluggishness when circulation becomes poor leaves you down in the dumps? Get rid of the blues and add zest to your working spirits with a cider stimulant that produces instant results.

Take half a cup of freshly shredded horseradish, the same measure of grated onion, and a quarter cup each of finely diced garlic and ginger, adding a spoon of powdered cayenne in a fairly large-sized jar. Pour sufficient apple cider vinegar to cover the herbal mix by about three inches. Keep the sealed jar in a warm place and allow it to steep for up to four weeks, ensuring to shake the contents to encourage proper mixing. Once the infusion is perfected, strain the herbs and add slightly warmed honey and apple cider vinegar. The resulting tonic should taste spicy, with a sweetish flavor tingling with warmth. At this stage, you can try flavoring the mix in any way you desire. Cinnamon, fresh turmeric root and lemon add a spicier flavor. Refrigerating the mix helps it last for longer periods. Consume a small shot daily as an invigorating tonic. It will do wonders to stimulate your appetite, keep the immune system fine-tuned and improve blood circulation.

A word of caution

The cider stimulant should be avoided if you're on medication for hypertension. If you are still tempted to try the tonic discontinue the tonic if you feel symptoms of excessive body warming and increasing tension.

Using cider stimulant herbs to create chutney

You may notice that the spent herbs of the cider stimulant are too tasty to be discarded. Don't worry, you can reuse the strained herbs and create fine chutney that will come in handy on a cold wintery day. Blend the used cider to paste adding warm honey, cayenne and grated walnuts, chopped raisins and dates. The resulting coarse paste should be delightfully pungent and sweet to taste. It adds a punch to rice, vegetarian dishes, and soups.

The herbal vitality syrup that fires the passion

Add half a spoon each of dried muira, eleuthero and maca herbs to two quarts of water in a pan and bring the mix to a simmering heat leaving a slight gap when you place the lid over the pan. Remove from the burner and add damiana, horny goat weed and milky oats, leaving the mix in a tightly sealed container overnight. The following day, strain the herbs through a sieve covered with muslin cloth. Simmer the mix adding two cups of honey slowly and within ten minutes you'll get a thick mix. At this stage, add a cup of fruit concentrate and half a cup of brandy. Cool and refrigerate the mix, taking two to four spoons daily. The refrigerated mix can be consumed over a three to four-month period.

Ayurvedic Chyawanprash made at home

Chyawanprash is a famous Ayurvedic formula that aids digestion, strengthens immunity and improves vitality, besides also acting as a strong aphrodisiac. It is so delicious that you'll be tempted to dip into the jar more often than necessary. An inexpensive way to enjoy the benefits of this wonderful ancient formula is to prepare it at home.

In an open bowl mix one part each of ashwagandha, eleuthero powder, maca, and Rhodiola powder, adding half a spoon cinnamon, a quarter spoon of ginger, and a pinch of cardamom powder. Now add a cup of raw honey, rose water and any fruit concentrate. Mash the ingredients to form a thickened paste and store it in the refrigerator. You can take one spoon of the paste twice daily straight from the container or by adding to warm water or tea. Alternatively, you can use cocoa powder to create dry balls of the thick paste wrapping the balls in parchment paper.

A ginseng recipe to beat them all

Ginseng, both the American and Asian variety, is well known for healing and rejuvenating properties, particularly the boosting of vitality and curing of sexual dysfunction. A honeyed recipe of ginseng would be just what the doctor ordered to boost sagging performance. You can use ginseng both as a freshly chopped root and in its dried or powdered form. Make sure it's finely chopped or shredded and then mix it with a generous helping of raw honey. Ensure to warm the honey before mixing and allow the mix to settle in a tightly sealed jar for up to three weeks. You should keep adding ginseng until you achieve a pasty thickness. A spoonful of matured honeyed ginseng can be consumed daily as a tonic for immune or reproductive system ailments and for promoting good health.

The refreshing cup of Asian tea or chai

For this recipe, you need three heaps of cinnamon, one tablespoon each of ashwagandha and eleuthero, half a spoon of dried ginger, one spoon of licorice root extract, along with two spoons of crushed cardamom, about 8 to 10 black whole peppercorns, and four cloves. When you prepare these herbs, ensure that they are dry, sifted and shredded coarsely but preferably not in powdered state as that leaves a residue. Mix these herbal ingredients well and store in an airtight jar.

To prepare the tea, add two spoons of the herbal mix to two cups of water in a pan raised to simmering heat over fifteen minutes. After removing from the heat add four spoons of black tea leaves. Allow the tea to steep in the mix for four to five minutes. At this stage, warm honey can be added. If you like a milky taste you can add warm milk to top off the tea sprinkled with powdered cinnamon, cocoa or nutmeg for a tangy taste. People on medication for high blood pressure would be advised not to add licorice to the herbal ingredients.

A kava love potion

Kava has this awesome reputation for stimulating sensuousness and keeping you stress-free and relaxed. Lovers the world over swear by this concoction and your sex life would be vastly improved by consuming kava. The kava chai or tea is a must-have in your herbal repertoire.

Take one cup of dried kava, a quarter cup of dried ginger, a quarter cup of cinnamon chips, a pinch of cardamom powder and whole black peppercorns, three cloves, and two chopped vanilla beans. Mix the herbs in two gallons of water and bring it to a gentle simmer keeping it on the burner for about four hours. Keep simmering till the flavor of kava comes out strongly. Then remove from the burner and add two cups of coconut milk (around 28 ounces) and leave the mixture to cool overnight in a closed container. Next morning, strain the mixture and sweeten to honey flavored with vanilla extract.

A note of caution

Excessive kava intake is known to be unsafe for the liver, and it isn't recommended if you're suffering from depression or hypertension. To err on the side of caution ensure to limit intake to 12 ounces daily. To add zing to kava chai, you can add a quarter cup each of ashwagandha, eleuthero, and Rhodiola.

The marvel of ginseng

Male libido got a much-needed boost on discovering the potency and resilience of Ginseng. This is an herb that not only restores sexual appetite and performance but also increases stamina by infusing energy when and where it matters.

To begin with, you need to choose a ginseng root that is fully matured and fresh. The best infusions are made using the well-known ginseng cooker which is a double lidded ceramic pot, one placed on top of the other. Ginseng root is covered in water in the upper pot while water simmers in the lower chamber. Six to eight hours of simmering on a low flame ensures the best ginseng root extraction. Then remove from the burner and allow the boiler pot to cool overnight without removing the root.

The tea can be consumed in small quantities throughout the day, taking care to eat sparingly and not overload your tummy on the day prior to the day after taking the tea. This elementary precaution guarantees that you enjoy the best health benefits of ginseng.

Traditional herbalists insist that strong ginseng tea is not a product fit for daily consumption. Rather, the best method is to undertake a fast for at least three days prior to taking the infused tea and to do this once in six months. But pairing ginseng with food is a great idea. Ginseng root can be added to a variety of soups, broths, curries, and wine to release its full medicinal value.

The male herbal recipe for combatting exhaustion

Combine two heaps of hawthorn berries, two parts of lemon balm, two measures of milky oats, two measures of nettle leaf and roots, along with hibiscus and horny goat weed. Make sure the herbs are freshly cut, sifted and shredded but not powdered, and store the mixture in a sealed jar. Then prepare an infusion on the same lines as we have explained previously. Take three to four cups of the brew daily to combat work-related stress and blues.

Hawthorn berries are renowned for relaxing and calming the mind and body and offer excellent protection against depression and anxiety. If you are habituated to yoga and other such healing sciences, herbal remedies produce really astonishing effects.

The art of bathing in an herbal ambiance

It is wisely said that a shower cleans the body, but a bath clears the mind, soothes the soul, and invigorates the spirit. The holistically healing power of an herbal bath has to be experienced to be fully appreciated. You may need to invest around twenty minutes preparing the herbal tea and readying the bath, but over time it will become a ritual as easy as breathing.

The sensationally sensual herbal bath

If you're exploring a new relationship or adding zest to the existing one, there's nothing to beat a sensuous bath with ingredients that will tantalize the senses. In a fresh warm (not too hot) bath, soak a handful of fresh rose petals and sage, along with three to four crushed cardamom pods, and a quarter spoon of powdered nutmeg. If you're wary of encountering the herbs directly, tie the herbs in a fine muslin bag attached by a thread to the nozzle of the tub, and expose the herbal sachet to a steady stream of warm water. At this stage as the tub gradually fills up add a few drops of clary sage or better still cardamom essential oil which imparts a pleasant scent to the bath.

The best herbal bath for relaxing sore muscles and a tired body

Gather two heaps each of eucalyptus and sage, adding four measures of Epsom salts to which you introduce around eight drops of rosemary or pine essential oil.

The early morning wake me up bath

Two parts each of rosemary and peppermint combined with essential oil of peppermint or geranium will do wonders to stimulate your body to peal physical condition.

The ultimate herbal relaxing bath

Chamomile tea is a popular relaxing drink for people experiencing sleep disturbances, but have you ever thought of including chamomile in your herbal bath? Pamper yourself with a deeply satisfying chamomile bath and a glass of rich red raised in one hand. The ingredients are two measures each of chamomile and sage along with one part each of hops and lavender, tempered with around eight drops of clary sage or vetiver essential oils.

Men's herbal healing recipes for common health problems

A vast and wonderful cornucopia of herbs is nature's bounty at your ready disposal for curing and healing a variety of common health issues. Experiment with these herbs and find out for yourself how you can aid the body in finding the right cure for each ailment. Your journey of discovery of herbal healing power begins right here.

Core issues we face in tackling men's health problems

More than women, men exhibit the woeful tendency to ignore or sideline important symptoms and indications of failing health. Feeling good is nice and feeling great and to be in good spirits is most welcome, but when you are down and out mentally, physically and spiritually there's not a moment to be wasted in procrastination. It's important to realize that a bruise or wound or even a rash won't disappear by themselves if left untreated. Men cannot afford to neglect or delay medical intervention when the body sends warning signals of what could be a deeper underlying health issue. The extremely intricate science of herbal healing awakens the body's inner resources and boosts its self-healing power like no other over the counter medical prescription. With herbs (skillfully and judiciously used) there are fewer side effects, and lasting good health is what men should aim for.

This is not to say that herbs offer the ultimate in healing capabilities and should comprise your entire treatment; on the contrary, a judicious mix of allopathic practices and herbal remedies does wonders to augment the body's healing impulse.

Male menopause

Starting in the mid-40s and progressing rapidly into the 50s, men undergo a physiological transformation marked by declining testosterone production. Reducing hormone levels play out with discernible psychological disturbances in this period cumulating in male menopause or andropause as it is now referred to as. The issue is that the male psyche, overburdened by age-old conceptions of virility and strength, is not conducive to self-analysis and self-healing. Men are less likely to discuss their health problems fearing that they'll be perceived as being weak. The gradual decline in testosterone results in irritability, sexual dysfunction, sexual inactivity and inability to conceive offspring. Sometimes, hair loss, sleep disturbances, and weight gain accompany these changes. The inability to come to terms with physical or psychological changes may lead to depression and anger that impact interpersonal relationships at home and office. Behaviorally, men may tend to live in denial but need to recognize that they are subject to cyclical hormonal changes that can devastate health if remedial measures are not initiated early on.

Combating age-related declining testosterone levels

From a high of 1000 Nanograms in the flush of youth to a low of 200 Nanograms in the seventies, testosterone declines at a steady pace, the decline speeding up after the 50s. To be sure, male menopause isn't a disease but a cyclical change that is best tackled with healthy variations in one's diet, exercise, and mood. Erectile dysfunction, slowing libido, anxiety, and cardiac issues usually characterize this phase but these problems are by no means irremediable.

Herbs transform male endocrine function

Men need a healthy endocrine system that smoothly balances levels of essential hormones and promotes overall good health, and herbs play a vital role in improving endocrine function. The following herbs are recommended as they are very safe and free from side effects.

Herbs that restore and enhance testosterone levels

500 mg capsules of Tribulus or Eleuthero taken twice each day for a month give a much-needed boost to hormone

levels in men. Stop the medication for at least a week between each monthly intake, ensuring not to exceed six months of treatment annually.

Prostatitis and prostatic cancer have an excellent antidote in nettle root which paves the way for a smoother reinvigoration of the male reproductive system. Follow the same dosage as for Tribulus and Eleuthero.

Rhodiola is another herb that restores depleting energy levels and boosts libido in men. Use the same dosage as with the earlier herbs.

Ashwagandha (following the same daily intake) is another miracle herb in Ayurvedic science that restores depleted sexual energy and combines well with the herbs we have already listed.

One teaspoonful of powdered maca root taken twice daily does wonders in boosting stamina and in ensuring that the male reproductive system functions without a glitch.

 Two 60 ml capsules of Ginkgo taken twice daily are good for improving memory. A prominent side effect of ginkgo is that it improves blood circulation in the penis, paving the way for improved penile e erection and sexual performance.

Milky oats would be of particular interest to men in stressful careers that adversely impact libido. Milky oats blended with a fine decoction of hawthorn, lemon balm, and St. John's wort does wonders in combatting stress-related sexual disorders.

Androstenedione, testosterone, dehydroepiandrosterone, and androsterone formulations that are synthetically prepared have a bioavailable substitute that is much safer – Pine pollen powder. The recommended dosage is one tablespoon of pollen powder taken in the evening that promotes sexual vigor and enhances erectile function. But this should not be taken over a prolonged period and should be used only to augment healthy body functions.

The disadvantages of testosterone replacement therapy (TRT) and bio-identical hormone replacement therapy (BHRT)

Both TRT and BHRT have been relatively successful in treating male sexual disorders but accompanied by a slew of harmful side effects. Herbs are a safer alternative that works gently in the background minimizing or completely doing away with side effects as they help the reproductive system grow stronger.

Healthy herbal potency enhancing solutions

This is a formulation that never ceases to amaze men as it improves their sexual vigor and stamina without having to deal with harmful side effects. Prepare a tincture using 2 spoons of Tribulus, and 1 spoon each of eleuthero, nettle root, and Rhodiola. The recommended dosage is one spoon of the tincture consumed thrice daily for a maximum period of one month followed by a week's rest. This herbal formulation is a safer alternative to standard TRT and BHRT therapy.

What men should avoid

Hops, a vital ingredient in beer (sorry to disappoint you guys), is a depressant that inhibits neurotransmission and which slows down sexual functioning. So if you are a habitual beer guzzler try varieties that do not contain hops. You can add licorice root, black cohosh, and vitex to your list of must avoid testosterone inhibitors that break your libido.

A note of caution in using herbal sex stimulants

Every individual responds differently to sexual stimulants so the safest practice is to monitor sexual health and performance closely while taking herbs and to discontinue herbs that are doing you harm not good.

Herbal energy balancing formulations

You may not have the time or resources to keep formulating tinctures, teas, and infusions on a daily basis and it may be cumbersome to carry them with you when you travel. If you are the constantly moving type, it's better to make a powder of the following essential herbs, paving the way for a quick fix booster when energy levels plummet during the day.

Mix one spoon each of ashwagandha, eleuthero, maca powder and pine pollen powder and store in a tightly sealed glass jar away from direct sunlight. You can also use opaque bottles that filter out UV light. One teaspoon of the mix consumed twice daily is a great energy booster.

The chocolaty herbal concoction to die for

If you have a fondness for sweet stuff, you'll love this dark chocolate candy spiced with fresh ginger and turmeric.

First of all, gather these ingredients; one cup of finely grated walnuts, a quarter cup each of Rhodiola powder, eleuthero powder, maca powder, and pine pollen powder, and one teaspoon each of vanilla extract and ground black pepper powder. To this mix add a spoon of sea salt and a cup of freshly grated ginger.

Separately, in the upper pot of a double boiler combine two cups of finely broken chunks of dark chocolate and half a cup of virgin coconut oil. Bring water to a boil in the lower pot and reduce the flame to low/medium to keep the water on simmer. Keep stirring the upper pot till the chocolate and coconut oil are smoothly combined. Now remove from the burner and add the rest of the ingredients stirring slowly till you get a gooey texture. At this stage, you can pour the mix into a chambered candy tray and allow the mix to cool at room temperature. Once the candy is firm you can separate the chunks and store in a tightly sealed container in the fridge. Just one or two helpings of this excellent candy will ensure that your hormone levels stay balanced throughout the day.

Tinea pedis, also known as Athlete's foot

This is a fungal infection that locates itself in the grooves between your toes and is an affliction plaguing men more than women. It creates a scaly, itchy skin that could dry and open up painful fissures that smell strongly. If you're not careful, the infection can spread to other parts of the body. Prevention is possible by keeping your feet clean and dry, by changing socks repeatedly, and by wearing sandals and shoes limiting exposure to the ground.

The best herbal remedy is a thick poultice of a black walnut hull. Allow at least three days to tackle the infection, and avoid socks and shoes to prevent staining. Chaparral and goldenseal are equally effective. You can also apply a diluted solution of apple cider vinegar though there may be a temporary burning sensation. Tea tree oil, myrrh, and thuja are other remedies.

The following remedies are very effective in combatting fungal infections

The herbal foot bath

Heat sufficient quantity of water in a pan and transfer to a wide-bottomed bucket used specifically for soaking the feet. Then add around 20 drops of tea tree oil, myrrh, and thuja essential oil, along with one cup of apple cider vinegar, mixing in a cup of olive oil. At this stage, the heated water will start emitting a strong fragrance. Then introduce your feet in the water and enjoy the warm tingling sensation as the herbs start working on the infection over a short span of ten to twenty minutes. After soaking, pat dry the feet using disposable tissue or fine muslin cloth which must be discarded after each use to prevent infection from spreading.

The herbal powder application

For busy men with little time for a wet soak, the herbal powder provides a faster and more convenient alternative. Mix half a cup of white clay with two tablespoons of chaparral powder, one spoon of black walnut hull powder, and one spoon of goldenseal root powder taken in a glass container. To the mix add a teaspoon of tea tree oil. Whisk thoroughly and allow the mix to mature for a couple of hours in the closely sealed jar. Sprinkle the powder generously on to a brush applicator and apply gently over the infected area. Take care not to insert the applicator into the herbal mix. The results will cheer you up in no time but for the darkish stains that may last a couple of days.

The herbal ointment

Fungal infections thrive in the warm and moist areas between toes, and it catches on especially after strenuous workouts and sports activities. Once the feet are cleaned and dried thoroughly, it's the best time to apply a powerful salve.

Using the upper pot of a double boiler, mix one tablespoon of black walnut hull powder, one tablespoon of dry chaparral powder, one tablespoon of organic goldenseal powder. Then blend with a cup of warm olive oil and add twenty drops of thuja, myrrh, and tea tree essential oil.

Bring the bottom pot full of water to a boil and then slow down to a gentle simmer. Allow the herbal mix to infuse the olive oil in the upper pot. Do this for not more than an hour. Allow the herbal mix to cool and let the residue settle at the bottom before straining the solids. You can drape cheesecloth over the strainer to keep out leftover particles. Next, slowly add a quarter cup of beeswax to the herbal oil in the pan gently warmed over a low burner.

Within a few minutes, you'll see the wax melting and the herbs gaining a thicker pasty texture. The cooled mixture can be preserved in a sealed jar ready for instant use.

You can apply the salve whenever it's convenient for you and when your feet can be rested for a couple of minutes. Applying the salve twice a day would be ideal for tackling any fungal infection.

Worries and anxieties

Anxiety attacks men, especially in the office set up. Such attacks become more frequent when men suffer their 'mid-life crisis' or menopause. The periodical hormonal imbalances and lowering levels of testosterone combine to aggravate moods. When anxiety becomes chronic, depression sets in. At this stage what men urgently need is good medication-assisted by helpful therapy and proper counseling to regain their positive mood. Herbs, men will be happy to know, provide a rich warehouse of nutrient-dense, energy-boosting, and mood-enhancing remedies.

Most men would be well aware that a depressive mindset makes them turn to the comfort of food. A proper diet is, therefore, a key rejuvenator when mind and mood suffer. Ideally, at such times the diet must be rich in nutrients, B vitamins, calcium, and omega fatty acids. Stimulants such as caffeine, food additives, and preservatives and colors fray the nerves and increase blood pressure further pushing men to the edge.

The herbal stress and anxiety busters

Soothing tonics that restore and revitalize

Some of the most powerful sedatives that nature provides are milky oats, passionflower, valerian, skullcap, and California poppy. Two cups of these invigorating tonics stem anxiety and prevent you from sinking into depression. They're excellent for restoring lost sleep patterns.

The relaxing valerian tincture

Valerian is noted for its powerful ability to fight depression but one needs to assess how the body reacts to this herb. If no side effects are noticeable, permit yourself a minute dose of valerian tincture on an hourly basis till the dark mood lifts.

The kava stress buster

A tincture of kava taken hourly through half teaspoons is an effective antidote to depression and anxiety attacks. But don't extend treatment beyond a week as it could affect liver function. The kava love potion or chai we described earlier is equally effective.

A stronger herbal therapy combatting depression

Fortunately for mankind, nature has stocked us with wondrous herbs that do great service in combating depression, the chronic and longer-lasting symptom of anxiety. Herbal power keeps nerves fighting fit, improves blood circulation and allays symptoms before anxiety becomes chronic.

The soothing ambiance of an herbal bath

A warm tub bath can be a rejuvenating experience in more ways than one. Firstly, the soak puts you in a relaxed frame of mind which gets boosted if you poise a glass of great wine in one hand. Secondly, the warm water unties muscular knots and relaxes your joints. Thirdly, the herbal ingredients present a soothing ambiance that heals you from the outside.

You could start by preparing a soothing tea out of lavender, sage, rosemary, oats, or chamomile, all of which have intense relaxing powers. Otherwise, you could add a few drops of essential oils directly into the warm water being careful not to overdo the dosage. A safer method is to pack the dry herbs into a tea bag or muslin cloth bag. This could be secured to the tub faucet, allowing warm water to trickle through the bag into the tub. After a while when you're relaxed in the tub you could release the tied bag into the water allowing its herbal contents to do their magic. A glass of wine and soothing lounge music complement this excellent relaxation routine. You'll love it, and don't be surprised if you find yourself repeating the routine every single day. On the practical side attempt an herbal bath every alternative day.

Imbibing the essence of flowery herbs

Go to your trusted herbalist and ferret out the floral essence that appeals to your senses. Inhaling a floral fragrance is a great way to enhance your mood and clear the cobwebs of depression. You really need to try this remedy to realize its instantaneous benefits.

Traditional herbs that beats depression hands down

St, John's Wort is globally renowned for its calming ability and has been an essential component of classical herbal cures. Read up on the herb to know if it's suitable for you, especially if you're being treated for existing medical complications. Its versatility is such that one can combine it with oats, lemon balm, and passionflower for added effect.

Milky oats, the electric green topping of the oats plant is excellent for combatting fatigue and chronic depression.

Passionflower is hugely appreciated for calming and toning up the central nervous system. It can be taken in the same herbal combination as with St. John's Wort and is recommended for men who have difficulty sleeping.

Valerian is highly recommended for hyperactive men who have trouble getting a good night's sleep. But use it with care if you are already on medication for high blood pressure and heart disease.

Damiana tackles depression by balancing the hormonal changes that occur in a man's body, especially in midlife amidst a stressful work environment.

Ginseng is an all-round health rejuvenator that has been the subject of much clinical evaluation. As with all other antidepressants, use the herb carefully, noting the subtle and not so subtle changes taking place in your body.

The problem with beer-guzzling

Beer, though a hot favorite among men, especially on hot summer days is unfortunately not what the doctor ordered for depression. Hops the key ingredient of beer, interferes with penile erection and general libido, and may even boost depression.

The tea/ tincture antidote for depression

A strong tea prepared using one portion each of hawthorn berries, lemon balm, milky oats, and St John's wort gives you an instantaneous pick up if you're suffering from depression, drooping spirits, grief or anger. The recommended dosage is two cups of tea daily or a spoon of tincture twice daily for a maximum period of one month.

Combatting vitamin D deficiency

Nowadays it is possible to get yourself medically tested for vitamin D deficiency. The scarcity of this crucial vitamin can affect blood circulation, nervous disorders, and immune system problems. The cheapest and most effective remedy is to ensure you get a dose of early morning sunshine every day. Alternatively, supplement your diet with vitamin D tablets of around 60000 IU every fortnight.

Don't neglect to exercise the body

The body like any finely tuned machine needs regular maintenance and nothing beats regular exercise or brisk walking. Being surrounded by nature uplifts the spirits as much as it heals the body.

Omega-3 Essential Fatty Acids (EFAS)

As we continue consuming the wrong type of foods, our tissues fill up with elements called free radicals that tear down cell walls. Over a period of time, this large scale destruction presents itself as disorders, disease, and inflammation. Omega fatty acids are substances naturally present in good foods that combat free radicals and restore the health of our immune system, nervous system, and circulatory system. If you're a meat-eater, try regular helpings of sardines, salmon and tuna. If you're a vegan add a good dose of flaxseeds, hemp seeds, and chia seeds to your daily diet.

Raising your serotonin levels

You may be making a serious mistake reaching for prescription antidepressants to combat sleep disorders and anxiety. The problem you may be facing is a sharp drop in serotonin levels. This is a chemical used in the brain and nervous system for impulse transmission. Low levels induce restlessness, anxiety, and depression in men. The healthier alternative is taking 5-hydroxytryptophan (5-HTP) supplements. The effects will be immediately felt through lowered irritability, fewer mood swings, and improved sleep. The maximum recommended dosage is 100mg thrice daily for a short of two weeks. It'd be better if you keep your doctor in the loop when taking these supplements.

S-adenosyl-L-methionine

S-adenosyl-L-methionine may sound like a mouthful. You can use the word SAME. This is a byproduct of liver metabolism. You need this element for maintaining a healthy nervous system, immune system, and skeletal system. Taking a SAME supplement will give you two essential benefits; it lowers pain and elevates your mood. You are safe with a smaller dose (200 mg twice daily) but do consult a doctor before increasing supplementation.

The sunshine vitamin

If you're regularly consuming milk and dairy products, and cod liver oil, you can be reasonably sure that your Vitamin D requirement is taken care of. But if this is not the case, and you are not exposing yourself to regular bouts of healing sunshine, you could be seriously deficient in this crucial vitamin. Vitamin D as D3 is the easiest that our bodies can absorb. Too little of the vitamin and too much of it are both dangerous so visit your physician who'll prescribe the right dosage after testing you for deficiency. But if you're confident of getting twenty minutes of daily sunshine you needn't bother with Vitamin D supplementation.

Mood elevating essence of flowers

The gentlest and most magical treatments an herbalist can prescribe for men is the floral essence Floral essences assist the body in correcting hormonal imbalances and conquer emotionally negative attitudes. They unlock our spiritual pathways. Just a tiny drop of the essence under the tongue is all that is needed to power a healing reaction. Clinical studies confirm that floral essences really work on improving moods and in allaying anxiety. The beauty of floral therapy is that they work on the same principles of homeopathy, where tiny doses diluted manifold increase the potency of the curative effect. As small a quantity as three to four drops of the essence of a flower is enough, consumed thrice daily, to work wonders on our damaged tissues.

The versatility of floral essences can be judged from the following table:

Agrimony: Calms the hyperactive mind, releasing positive vibrations that enhance our moods. This is an excellent remedy for suppressed emotions that damage us from within.

Aspen: Great for relief from uncontrolled apprehensions, fears, and feelings of diffidence.

Cherry plum: Effective for seeking relief from chronic hypertension and nervous breakdowns.

Elm: This is very effective for men dealing daily with work-related tensions and onerous deadlines that endanger a feeling of being overwhelmed.

Gentian: Especially effective for overcoming depression brought on by so-called failures or setbacks in life.

Hornbeam: Excellent remedy for fighting weariness and exhaustion brought on by the grinding routine of daily life.

Impatiens: For men perpetually on a short fuse that feels irritated at the slightest provocation.

Larch: For overcoming diffidence and the fear of the unknown that prevents men from realizing their immense potential.

Mimulus: A wonderful flower that releases positive energy needed to accomplish challenging tasks.

Mustard: Excellent for men prone to manic depression and which encourages the desire to excel.

Olive: This is an excellent remedy for amnesia and compensates for depleted energy levels.

Pine: The ice breaker promising freedom from repressed emotions and fast failures that prevent men from moving on with their lives.

Star of Bethlehem: Great for releasing men from the vice-like grip of past traumatic experiences.

Sweet chestnut: Promises absolute freedom from the agony of enforced loneliness and the desolation it produces in men.

Wild rose: Freeing men from the inability to enjoy life to the full and energizing the day with an elevated mood.

Floral essences offer safe cures without the side effects produced by modern drugs. These essences lay the foundation for a healthier integration of our mental, physical and spiritual worlds. The most effective results are guaranteed when you combine meditation, yoga and physical exercise with floral therapy. It is wisely said that depression is a window of opportunity nudging a man to explore alternative therapies that make a huge difference to his wellbeing. Depression is nothing but an indication that man is rejecting his inner voice that is prompting him to take a path that is more in tune with nature.

Leveraging herbs to combat male urinary tract issues

Advancing age invariably produces complications in the male urinary tract, and it's usually the bladder and prostate gland that are the root cause of the conflict. Cystitis is a common condition affecting the urinary bladder that produces a burning and painful feeling while urinating. The second most common issue men face is prostatitis, an inflammation in the prostate gland.

There excellent and safe herbal remedies that'll help you clear these symptoms within two to three days:

Teas: The best known herbal remedies for urinary tract infection are uva urvsi, buchu, cleavers, marshmallow root, chickweed, nettle, and dandelion leaf. Two to three cups daily of a tea made out of three or more of these herbs are an excellent antidote for restoring urinary health.

Tinctures: A concentrated tincture of Echinacea taken at least thrice daily brings down infection and boosts the immune system thereby preventing the problem from recurring.

The combination tincture: Taking a combination of tinctures of goldenseal and Echinacea (half a teaspoon) at least thrice daily will cure the worst infections giving you a new lease of life.

Saw palmetto: Is known to impact the prostate gland beneficially and is also very effective in reducing inflammation in a cystitis attack.

Preventing bacterial infection: Cranberry juice taken in three cupfuls evenly dispersed through the day helps clear infections fast. The best variety is the unsweetened version which can be mixed with apple juice for a delicious twist.

Lemon: Prepare a quart of water mixed with the juice of one whole lemon adding a drop of uva ursi tincture to create a powerful inflammation fighter. The water can be evenly consumed throughout the day and will ease the discomfort of urination.

Combine these simple herbal remedies with lots of rest and relaxation, and for added comfort place a hot water bottle over the kidney area to soothe irritation. It will also help if you refrain from sexual encounters until the urinary tract infection clears. Also avoid alcohol, meaty dishes and spices that tend to irritate the bladder and produce acidic urine.

The best herbal formulation to attack cystitis

Simple herbal alternatives that give you permanent relief from chronic cystitis:

1.	Prepare a tea combining two heaps of uva ursi, and one portion each of buchu, cleavers and marshmallow root. Three cups of the strong tea taken thrice daily for three to four days clears up the worst attacks of cystitis.

2.   A tincture of the very same herbal combination will take you at least a month to prepare and mature. This is the recommended route if bladder problems are common to you. A quarter teaspoon taken hourly from morning to sundown for three consecutive days ought to clear your distress.

Sores or inflamed condition of penile foreskin

The foreskin covering the glans or head of the male penis poses problems across all age groups. The problem arises when excessive moisture combines with bacterial growth to encourage infections. This may lead to itching soreness and pain when the foreskin is retracted. The preventive measure is to shower and clean the genital areas frequently and allow the area to dry thoroughly before donning undergarments. It also helps to wear comfortable loose-fitting cotton garments that absorb sweat and keep the genital area dry. Allopathic medication tends to be strong and may entirely dry out the penis withdrawing the lubrication between the foreskin and glans. Herbalists suggest excellent herbal remedies that can remedy this problem quietly and efficiently.

A powder made of two portions each of elm bark, and marshmallow, and one portion of goldenseal creating a slithery mix is very effective when sprinkled over the affected area twice daily. To keep from spoiling undergarments it's advisable to wrap the head of the penis in soft muslin cloth or cotton.

If powder application is cumbersome, you can brew a strong tea using a mix of two parts each of yarrow, calendula, and goldenseal. The tea can be used to wash the penis, especially its tip, leaving the penis to soak the healing tea for about 10 minutes. The time just after the shower or bath is most appropriate for soaking and drying.

Another soak that is equally powerful is a mix of two portions each of witch hazel bark, white oak bark, and raspberry leaf that can be used to gently wash the infected spot twice or thrice daily till the infection clears.

To boost healing it's better to consume more herbs orally. Mix two portions each of goldenseal, echinacea, marshmallow root, and myrrh powders and bind the mix in small capsular form. Adults can consume two capsules thrice daily, while children can be given half the dose twice daily.

If children are too small or unable to swallow capsules, the same remedy can be mixed to form a tincture. Half a spoon of the tincture can be administered orally every four hours till the infection clears.

To circumcise or not to circumcise is the question

In many parts of the world, kids are routinely circumcised just after birth or at a young age. America apparently beats the global trend with a large number of males leaving the hospital with their foreskin intact. Elsewhere, religious reasons and parental pressure ensure that circumcision is not a choice that the young male is allowed to take independently.

The advantages of retaining the male foreskin are many. The foreskin forms a protective cover over the sensitive glans or head of the penis. A tough but pliable foreskin not only protects the penis from physical injury; it also lubricates the glans and keeps it free of infection by secreting a whitish discharge. All it needs is to be physically retracted to enable the head of the penis to be cleaned thoroughly at least once daily, not to mention the regular change of undergarments. A retained foreskin carries sensitive nerve endings that heighten pleasure during the sex act.   In fact, this is probably the sole reason why ultra-conservative societies encouraged circumcision and gave it a religious halo. So, the arguments favoring retention of the male foreskin weigh strongly against the need for circumcision.

The ache that benumbs male patients and causes loss of millions of man-hours

Billions of dollars are spent annually in the search for an allopathic sure for the common headache. It's an open secret that over the counter remedies in America have created a multibillion-dollar industry which sometimes does far more harm by way of side effects. Headaches may be transitory, or they may sometimes develop into a more chronic form. Headaches are mainly due to stress and overwork, lack of sleep and improper diet. Constriction of arteries in the brain and excessive blood pressure are other factors. If you study your headache you may notice that it usually accompanies fatigue, exhaustion, and emotional distress. Before even attempting medication, it would be wiser to try and root out the underlying cause. In any case, it's not a problem that deserves to be ignored or routinely suffered hoping that it will simply go away. A remedy is a must, but you're safer if you turn to herbs.

Repetitive headaches

If headaches keep reappearing at regular intervals, you need to closely study what you're eating and your immediate surroundings. It's possible that a food allergen might be triggering the ache, or smoke, dust and pollen particles might be causing the headache. It's equally possible that you may be suffering from digestive upsets brought on by an improper diet.

Aches emanating within the circulatory system

Excessive acidity brought on by overconsumption of alcohol, carbonated beverages, and cold and acidic foods can affect blood circulation creating vascular headaches. The immediate remedy should be taking something that quickly alkalizes the body and reduces acidity.

Stress aches

A disturbed and hyperactive mindset can create recurring headaches. One of the best ways of judging the root cause is to reassess what you consumed and what your mind was engaged with prior to and after the attacks occur. Emotional strain, excessive salt intake, lack of water in the body, and low blood sugar can trigger headaches. Try rehydrating the body with water mixed with the juice of a freshly squeezed lemon. Cranberry juice or diluted raw apple cider vinegar are excellent pick me ups. Freshly brewed teas of chamomile, skullcap, and passionflower produce a calming effect. Sometimes, the best solution is to take a break from what you've been doing and to take a re4freshing walk in the park or to simply switch your thoughts to a meditative mode.

Herbs can be your best friends in overcoming debilitating headaches.

Relaxing your feet

Soak your tired feet in a tub of hot water mixed with healing herbs. Keep yourself occupied with a glass of chamomile tea or a warm decoction of St. John's wort. Get your companion to hold an ice pack to the nape of your neck or do a gentle messaging of the shoulder muscles. If you want to boost the relaxing powers of chamomile tea simply add a quarter spoonful of valerian tincture to the tea.

Boosting your vitamin intake

Men battling sugar problems can do with an extra shot of vitamins. Niacinamide, a vital ingredient in the B-complex family of vitamins, is known to break headaches effectively if taken in 100 mg capsules thrice daily.

Acidity and its herbal panacea

If an acidic environment is wreaking havoc in your digestive system, the best antidote is to attempt a gentle alkalizing herbal mix that restores the pH balance in the blood. The Japanese are fond of consuming salted plums and miso soup which happen to be very effective alkalizers. If salted plums are unavailable try salted olives; they're just as effective.

The age-old herbal tonic called the Swedish Bitter is very helpful in neutralizing acidic secretions in the digestive system.

The common lemon is a readily available digestive especially if you habituate yourself to consuming a glass of freshly squeezed lime flavored with salt. It's tangy and tasty and relieves gastric upsets quietly.

Tackling stress-induced vascular headaches

Prepare a healthy decoction using dandelion root, burdock root and yellow dock root in descending order of proportions (three, two, one) adding a drop of valerian tincture to the mix. A quarter cup of this tea can be consumed on an hourly basis. The valerian tincture adds a sedative touch, completely relaxing you in no time at all.

Your best bet for soothing that tension headache

Prepare a strong brew composed of two portions of feverfew, and one part each of California poppy and lavender. For the poppy, try combining the plant leaf, flower, and seed for best results. Try a quarter cup of the brew every hour till you get the desired results – a calmer and pain-free head. For headaches that tend to repeat or become chronic, it's better to shift to a tincture using the same ingredients and measures. It will take you three to four weeks for the tincture to mature, but the end results will be worth the wait especially if you're a chronic sufferer.

For men that are exhausted by mental tension

The best method is to prepare an infusion using three portions (spoons) of chamomile, three spoons of lemon balm, and one part each of the passionflower and skullcap. Keep drinking at least half a cup of the delightful brew, on an hourly basis, till you get relieved of the headache.

Treatment of migraine headaches

Migraine tells us that somewhere within the body, the body's protective mechanisms are temporarily down till you find the root cause and take corrective action. Hormonal insufficiencies, food allergies, immune deficiency, and stress are common triggers, while pollutants, molds, and fungi are external factors. The problem with modern medicine is that you'll be grappling with the side effects as if the original problem was not bad enough. Subtle changes in diet and lifestyle besides a serious attempt at identifying the causative agent are helpful in combating chronic headaches.

Vitamin supplementation

300 mg daily of Niacinamide along with 200 mg each of rutin and vitamin B6 spread evenly in dosages throughout the day will combat migraines in most instances.

Another very effective remedy is vitamin C in even doses of 2000 mg taken twice daily along with half a spoon of guarana which gives you an extra special caffeine kick to elevate the mood. If you find that too strong a stimulant, kindly discontinue.

Talking of caffeine, it's OK to consume one or two cups of freshly brewed coffee or a simple tea of guarana extract or for that matter any other caffeinated herb to seek relief from migraine. The symptoms dissipate early leaving you soothingly refreshed.

The blended feverfew remedy for instant relief from migraine

Instead of taking remedial action after the onset of a migraine, try a soothing blend of feverfew that acts as a quietly efficient preventive care medication. Mix together two portions of feverfew along with one portion each of California poppy seed, lavender, and St. John's wort which presents you with a strong and mutually fine-tuned blend that attacks migraine slowly and steadily. Drink at least a quarter cup of the infusion every half hour when you suspect that migraine is coming on too strong. Men prone to migraine would do better to consume half a spoon of tincture mixed in warm water taken at least thrice daily till a feeling of calm pervades.

Tackling cardiac distress

The heart, our major blood-pumping organ, also happens to be the seat of our emotions if we believe what our ancestors say. That has more than a grain of truth because stress and improper diet can play havoc with our blood vessels layering them with heart-stopping cholesterol. Cardiac disease is a well-known silent killer that all men need to guard against particularly as they approach their mid-fifties. Men need to reduce stress which is often the biggest contributor to cardiac ailments. But the good news is that cardiac symptoms are the easiest to treat if we make subtle and not so subtle changes to our diets and attitudes towards workplace stress.

In treating cardiac problems it's important to address the symptoms early on.

You need to be alert to a mild to severe ache that troubles the chest. Carefully study your digestive reactions and bowel movements to rule out gastric disorders that most often create the very same symptoms.

The chest is not the only area that registers cardiac stress. It could materialize as a chronic headache, a sharp pain in the jaws or a radiating pain that crisscrosses the arms starting from the shoulder downwards.

If the heart is not pumping appropriately, it means that tissues are being deprived of oxygen, and this shows up as shortness of breath signally you to inhale deeply to compensate for the oxygen deprivation.

A sure sign of a slowing heart is the kind of anxiety that appears before your palms and body start sweating profusely for no reason at all. These are symptomatic of slowing blood circulation.

If the digestive system appears to be stressed it may indicate that poor circulation is impeding the proper digestion and assimilation of food.

A sudden sense of dizziness may indicate that the heart is not pumping sufficient blood to reach the brain. In some instances, this may be accompanied by nausea and vomiting.

Often extreme anxiety slows down the heart and the system tries to compensate by spasmodically increasing heartbeats which produces palpitating symptoms.

The difficulty lies in the fact that most of these symptoms may be simply stress-induced and temporary but you may need a clinical diagnosis to confirm whether you are becoming a heart patient.

Preventive measures to stay clear of cardiac disease

Diet is, of course, the most important measure that protects men from the onset of cardiac disease. You need to go easy on oils and fatty foods as you enter the fifties. Research heart-healthy oils and control your craving for strong curries and gravy laden foods, especially junk food. If you consume fats in excess of daily requirements it leads to the deposition of excess glycogen in the fatty tissue around the waist and thighs. The best antidote is to exercise at least twenty minutes daily in the mornings combining aerobics in the early hours with something less stressful like yoga and meditation in the evenings. Regular outdoor activity is not only a stress reliever but also paves the way for fat-busting in a big way.

Essentials for a heart-healthy lifestyle

Consume good quantities of fruits that are colorfully well endowed like blueberries and cranberries as that gives you a sufficient quantity of bioflavonoids which combats inflammation in heart tissue.

A healthy omega-3 fatty acid intake is assured if you introduce lots of fish into your diet, fish like salmon, tuna and sardines.

Lightly boiled or steamed dark green leafy veggies are your best source of antioxidants so ensure these veggies form an essential part of your daily food intake.

Avoid or drastically cut down the intake of red meat and switch to lean meat in the form of fish and chicken or protein-rich soya bean.

Oils like olive sunflower and hemp are better substitutes for rich butter and margarine. You'd be doing yourself a favor by reducing fried meats in a big way. Also, check oils for flavor and freshness before consumption.

Did you know that sugar stokes cancerous growth in the body even in apparently healthy men? Though sugar is essential to good health excessive consumption could encourage inflammation in tissues. So cut your sugar intake and avoid sugar substitutes because their effects are still not fully researched and understood.

The herbal path to a heart-healthy lifestyle

The beauty of herbal remedies is that they help relax you mentally, improve blood circulation and strengthen heart muscles. Some of the most important side effects are reduced cholesterol and lowered blood pressure. That's not bad for a side effect compared to what modern medicine delivers! (234)

Miracle herbal remedies for heart "burn"

Hawthorn

If there's a superstar in your herbal collection that mitigates heart disease most effectively it has to be Hawthorn, an immensely versatile herb. The herb is so packed with heart-healthy flavonoids that it easily rivals cherries, blueberries, grapes, and red wine. The immediate benefits are regularized heartbeat, improved circulation, and lower cholesterol levels. The herb is best consumed as a tonic mixed with pure honey, and that sounds delightful, doesn't it?

Garlic

Three raw cloves daily are all that your heart needs to function normally. If raw garlic is too overpowering, you could switch to capsules or liquids. A note of caution is to avoid garlic if you are prone to digestive upsets.

Ginkgo

This herb has an exalted place in herbal repertoire as an effective remedy for heart disease. Its action is predominantly on the thickness of blood and its circulation within the body. By decreasing the viscosity of blood it prevents blood from coagulating abnormally to form clots that bring on strokes. The herb also speeds up blood circulation significantly. This produces a side effect that will of great interest to men – it promotes the flow of blood into the penis and boosts erectile function. So now we have a single herb that not only improves heart health but also acts as a sexual power booster.

Cayenne hot chili pepper

Cayenne has been underestimated for its beneficial effect on the heart. It works predominantly by speeding up the flow of blood throughout the body. People unused to the chili pepper may notice a rosy tint to facial skin and a flushed appearance and kind of body warming associated with its action. A pinch of cayenne diluted in warm water mixed with honey is a great booster for the circulatory system ensuring that you breeze through the day in a healthy spirit.

Ashwagandha

This is an ancient Indian Ayurvedic herb we are already familiar with in this book. It plays a significant role in combating stress by relieving anxiety. That's great news for heart patients that are already facing repeated anxiety attacks. Ashwagandha is highly recommended in relieving symptoms of congestive heart failure.

What men need to know about cholesterol

Cholesterol is the news for all the wrong reasons, but that doesn't mean we can do without it.

If cholesterol was not essential to the production of a host of male and female hormones our sex lives would have taken a toss.

Without it vitamin D can't be synthesized, our immune system would be compromised, our nerves would suffer irreparable damage, our metabolism would come to a standstill and we would become sterile or infertile.

The liver uses cholesterol to produce bile which helps digest oils and fats.

Without the antioxidant effect of cholesterol-free radicals would damage cells and make us age faster.

The problem arises when blood carries excess cholesterol over long periods. This encourages the heavier (bad) cholesterol molecules to coat the arteries with a whitish plaque that impedes blood flow. This is how we get heart disease that leads to cardiac arrest.

Leveraging the best cholesterol controlling herbs

Artichoke, especially the leaves of the plant, encourages the liver and gall bladder to produce and store bile salts which aid digestion. Just half spoon of the tincture taken thrice dally is enough to control and regulate cholesterol production.

Grind milk thistle seed manually into a fine powder and sprinkle around half spoon on food before consumption. It has a strong antioxidant effect besides reducing high cholesterol levels within days.

Ingest three to four shiitake mushrooms daily for a week to reduce high cholesterol. You'll see a healthy 10 percent reduction in bad cholesterol levels. There are many associated health benefits to these wonderful mushrooms.

One of the best substitutes for modern medicine is Guggul, an Ayurvedic ancient Indian herbal remedy. Taking three capsules of 23 mg thrice daily for a week is enough to raise good cholesterol levels and stabilize your HDL/ LDL cholesterol ratio.

All these herbal remedies deliver better results than modern medicine without leaving painful side effects.

Controlling Hypertension

One of the biggest headaches that modern medicine has to deal with is hypertension, the raised blood pressure that constricted arteries face. The universally accepted fact is that this is a disorder that is chronic to societies that consume junk food in excess. Mediterranean and Eastern societies do not face a similar problem. So it boils down to diet and physical lifestyle that we choose. Excessive alcohol, tobacco smoking, and chewing and irregular dieting habits all contribute to increasing hypertension.

Ways to control hypertension

We usually end up consuming ten times more salt than our bodies are designed to take. Even though salt is essential for survival, too much of it can boost water retention. This makes our kidneys overwork and overloads the heart too.

An excellent remedy for lowering blood pressure is dandelion leaf which infuses potent levels of potassium which lowers and controls blood pressure and also cleanses the kidney without straining the heart.

The huge amount of beneficial organosulphur compounds in Garlic makes it an excellent remedy for sustaining healthy blood pressure levels. It also protects the heart.

In use since ancient times, motherwort dilates the arteries releasing the pressure on the heart and improves blood circulation. The tissues get oxygenated and vital nutrients reach organs faster. For a healthy overall calming and relaxing effect nothing beats this wonderful herb.

Linden flower ingested as a tonic has a soothing effect on the nervous system and also prevents palpitations and irregular heartbeat. It's best taken as a strong tea for relaxation.

Mistletoe has a direct effect on the vascular system easing the pressure on the heart by improving circulation. But, you need to take it in modest doses and that too under medical supervision as too much of it can prove toxic.

If you consume seeds of flax, primrose and black currant you get adequate inputs of fatty acids and the benefit of lots of fiber that keeps the digestive tract clear and healthy.

The natural cure for Herpes

Herpes is a sexually transmitted disease caused by a virus, and it's characterized by clusters of sores or blisters that swell and become painful. Even with modern medicine, the infection lasts for weeks creating acute discomfort.

Natural remedies seem to work faster and provide bigger relief.

Licorice root applied locally as a tincture is useful for drying up Herpes sores in no time. But the tincture can be strong so it's best diluted with water. Licorice can also be taken orally when the infection is severe. The only precaution is to avoid licorice altogether if you're suffering from high blood pressure or a heart condition.

Lemon balm applied externally as a cream or an ointment can be very effective in reducing the severity of herpes infection. It has a strong antiviral effect and is also a potent relaxing agent. You are advised against taking the essential oil orally as that could create problems for your thyroid gland.

The antiviral tincture blend ideal for herpes

Mix two portions of licorice root tincture and one portion each of calendula tincture and St. John's wort tincture for application locally. If necessary dilute the same tincture blend with water and take a teaspoonful thrice daily till you are completely cured.

Libido and declining sexual potency

Sexuality and sexual performance should worry men because not less than 30 million men in America report reduced sexual activity for various reasons. Roughly half of the men in the age group from 40s to their 70s experienced erectile dysfunction. The scenario is actually worsening because younger men reaching their 30s are now complaining of reduced sexual activity.

Following the introduction of Viagra in the market more than a million prescriptions were written, and the wonder drug was touted as the next best thing for male libido. But its side effects were sidelined. Viagra improved blood circulation to the penis creating a prolonged erection needed to complete coitus. But slowly and steadily, the side effects began to be noticed which included headaches, dizziness and raised blood pressure among other symptoms. What was missed in the dialogue was that Viagra did precious little to correct the underlying issue, which was impotency.

More than any issue it is the faulty lifestyle that we follow that is responsible for a malfunctioning reproductive system. Junk food, irregular sleeping habits, lack of nutrition, and a stressful work atmosphere are major red flags leading to the decline of male libido. Age is not as important a factor as is normally assumed. Both men and women leading healthy and productive lives are sexually very active past their fifties. An improved lifestyle is we urgently need to lead a healthier sex life.

Improve your exposure to regular exercise

If aerobics and a gym workout are beyond your abilities, try something simpler and stress-free like walking or light jogging, and strengthen and tone muscles using yoga and yogic postures. A daily dose of calm meditation does wonder to recharge spiritual power. Hegel exercises do wonders for strengthening the hips and promoting sexual performance. These exercises also improve the urinary system and the functioning of the prostate. These are two major areas that contribute to maximum maladies in male health if they are neglected.

Fresh air and fresh nutritious food

Our body eliminates tons of toxins on a daily basis and we can aid the body in a big way by improving outdoor activity. Lots of fresh air means improved oxygen intake and healthier lungs in addition to improved blood circulation – all vital for keeping tissues normal and healthy. On the nutritional front, we need to improve our intake of fresh fruit and vegetables and simultaneously reduce our dependence on meat giving more space to vegetarian sources of protein. Instead of popping vitamin pills, try sourcing natural vitamins that come from veggies and fruit which come bundled with powerful enzymes. Substitute caffeine with fruit and vegetable juices that not only assuage thirst but also provide natural fiber and the energy boost sufficient to carry you through a hard day's work.

Changing the daily shower routine

One of the best ways to improve stamina, vitality and sexual potency is to start and end the day with a slow and relaxing hot shower and cap it with a spray of cold water. It does wonders for improving blood circulation, a key factor in improving sexual performance.

The herbal remedy for libido enhancement

Longer lasting sexual activity and improved climax are achievable using herbal remedies that outdo Viagra without bringing on serious side effects. Herbs act fast by improving the production of male sex hormones that control and balance male libido. Palmetto offers excellent support to the prostate gland a key system that controls semen health. Take in healthy doses of ashwagandha, damiana, horny goat weed, maca, milky oats, and Rhodiola to boost reproductive health. These herbs are very powerful and stimulate sexual performance with sustained energy levels. Energy balls, maca balls, and root beer teas are excellent tonics that reinvigorate mood and boost sexual activity. Half a spoon of ginseng, that enormously beneficial wonder herb, acts as an instant pick-me-up for men of all ages. Instead of reaching out for cookies and crackers, consume just a quarter cup of pumpkin seeds and you'll get your daily boost of zinc which plays a very important supportive role in promoting reproductive health.

If there is one herb that closely mimics Viagra it is Yohimbe. It stimulates the central nervous system and causes blood vessels to dilate, bringing more blood and oxygen to penile tissue – a very important effect that is useful in bringing on and prolonging an erection. But this herb is so powerful that its use must be supervised by a qualified herbalist. Otherwise, you could open your system to vascular diseases and high blood pressure. Try avoiding formulations that source Yohimbe from the wild and instead shift to the herb that is cultivated organically on good soil.

Supplementing important vitamins and essential ingredients

Herbs that we have listed should not be used as quick-fix solutions for a one night stand. The best way to use these herbs is to follow a system of incremental dosage, sticking to a prolonged treatment period. This does wonders in promoting reproductive health and also helps in avoiding dangerous side effects.

Brazil nuts, coconuts, peanuts, oats and soybean foods give you plenty of the amino acid L-Arginine which helps build and repair reproductive cells.

Avocados, fish, cabbage, cauliflower, and almonds are a rich source of L-Choline, a crucial B vitamin component that is very effective in shoring up sexual arousal and performance.

Apples, bananas, and watermelon give you adequate doses of Vitamin B-6 which plays a big role in maintaining healthy male sex hormone balance.

With the passage of time, declining levels of zinc promote listlessness and declining libido. Garlic, sesame seeds, sunflower seeds, and seafood shore up the body's reserves of zinc making it possible to improve the quality and health of male sex cells.

Clinical research has now established that Vitamin D is essential not only to improved nerve and bone health but is also essential to reproductive health. So, waste no time in getting your fifteen minutes of glorious sunshine and go for healthy doses of seafood, sunflower seeds, oats, and quinoa.

The problem of male Infertility

Infertility refers to the problem of not being able to conceive healthy offspring because of diminished health and motility of the male sex cells or sperms. Unlike impotence, infertile males may produce healthy erections and may be very active sexually but their sperm lacks the power to produce offspring. The problem is common among sportsmen active in pursuits like cycling and horse-riding that increase pressure on the genital system. Imbalanced thyroid function may also destabilize the levels of testosterone causing men to lose erections and the appetite for sex. Herbs such as ginseng, eleuthero, Rhodiola, ashwagandha, nettles, and milky oats do wonders to stimulate sexual activity based on a healthier reproductive system.

The problem of sleeplessness or insomnia

More than a third of American males suffer from sleep disorders. You'll find these otherwise healthy men pacing the nights restlessly, depriving themselves of much-needed rest. The human body needs a regular dose of 8 hours of uninterrupted sleep to help detoxify the body. When that sleep cycle is disrupted, the result is anxiety, stress and emotional problems that come to the fore. A sleep-deprived body becomes worn out and lacks the energy to pursue daily tasks. Sleeping pills do more harm than good and they can become addictive if used over a period of time. The question is, why risk your health with modern medicine and therapies when there are herbs that do the work for without dangerous side effects.

The central nervous system and the adrenal glands can become exhausted through hyperactivity and are in dire need of rest even if that rest is enforced and doesn't come naturally. And you can trigger a natural resting response easily by using ashwagandha the power-packed Indian herb. Start by drinking one or two cups of the tea of ashwagandha during the day followed by a cup just before bedtime. The relaxing effect will astonish you.

A cup of warm and soothing chamomile tea is just what the herbalist orders for the chronic insomniac. It is as effective for children as it is for the seniors who become seriously sleep-deprived.

A strong tincture of equal portions of hops and valerian taken just before bedtime can ease stress, relieve anxiety, and soothe the nervous and digestive systems.

The tension and stress associated with muscularly active men can be eased considerably using half a spoon of the tincture of kava, repeating the dose for three consecutive hours before bedtime.

Two cups of strong skullcap tea consumed morning and evening are useful in calming the thinker and chronic worrier who suffers from sleep deprivation.

One of the safest remedies for insomnia happens to be a personal favorite – the valerian tincture. Take just one tablespoon of the tincture nearing your normal sleeping hour and wake up refreshed from a deep and soothing slumber.

When the muscles tear and the bones break

Muscular and skeletal problems are common not only to sportsmen but also to the daily workers that are consumed by physical activity. But many men, partly due to bloated egos, refuse to be slowed down by these problems, treating them as passing irritants. In many cases this results in irreparable damage to the tissues, creating problems that land the patient on the operating table. One such problem that plagues men of all ages is backache and lower leg pain. Light exercises and therapies involving stretching muscles may end up doing more harm than good in the long run.

By all means continue the therapies the doctor recommends but follow up with herbal treatments that restore muscular tone, revitalize sore ligaments, and strengthen tired tendons.

ST. JOHN'S WORT is an age-old remedy used frequently to remedy aches and repair nerve damage. The best remedies involve the fusion of fresh summertime flowers to form an oil best for external applications. For oral consumption, the best remedy is the concentrated tincture or strong tea.

Turmeric has established itself as an aggressive antioxidant that fights inflammation and cancer. Turmeric has a protective action against damages inflicted on bones, ligaments, and tendons. For men, it offers surefire protection against the onset of testicular, prostate and bone cancers. Turmeric tea prepared twice or thrice a day can be very refreshing and rejuvenating. If preparing a tea is laborious, try applying turmeric paste over affected areas of the skin and see the difference it makes.

The only irritation will be the persistence of a bright orange color which disappears in a couple of days. (271)

Cannabis - The most effective remedy for tackling inflammation and relieving pain

There may not be a plant that has been so systematically investigated and clinically tested than Cannabis, renowned for its anti-inflammatory and pain-relieving potency. Yet Cannabis continues to be discriminated against, continuing to be labeled as illegal in many states. What is little publicized about Cannabis is that it tackles inflammation and relieves pain with barely any side effects compared to pharmaceutical pain killers. What's more, the discomfort wears away faster when Cannabis is administered to the patient. Cannabis remains an effective antidote to even the most chronic symptoms of pain and neuromuscular inflammation.

The Epsom Salt Bath

You'd be surprised how effectively an Epsom salt bath soothes aches, relieves pain and rejuvenates sore muscles and tendons. The miracle lies in the ready absorption of magnesium through the skin which replenishes the body's reserves of this vital element. Stir a warm bath tubful of water with two cups of Epsom salt and enjoy a 30 minutes soak. If you are keen on using a salve of Epsom salt directly on to sore body parts keep the tub temperature moderately warm and not too hot.

The universally debilitating leg cramp

They'll tell you that a leg cramp isn't serious enough to cry all day about, but just one spasm is enough to make you miserable enough to question that logic. Low potassium levels or something leading to an electrolyte imbalance in the body is enough to throw muscles into spasms that tighten into painful knots, making even the slightest movement painful beyond words. Rubbing or messaging muscles might worsen the problem.

Apple cider vinegar is a fast-acting antidote to muscle stress and unties muscular knots faster than any pharmaceutical pain killer. Those prone to muscle cramps would do well to orally consume two parts of apple cider vinegar mixed with one part of clear raw honey, diluted in a cup of warm water. As a booster dose try applying and gently massaging a small quantity of the vinegar directly over the affected part. You'd be amazed how quickly the discomfort disappears.

To prevent recurrence of leg cramps try boosting your intake of apples and bananas, or mushrooms and potatoes, all of them excellent reservoirs of potassium. You could also ensure to consume good calcium cum magnesium supplement to augment body reserves of this vital element.

The best electrolyte replacement therapy happens to be the humble lemon. When you feel exhausted after the day's work or even when you are working out, walking or jogging, drinking a glass of freshly squeezed lemon diluted in clearwater is the ideal way of clearing the blues and rejuvenating the body.

Malignancy of the Prostate

The scary news is that around 30 to 35 percent of American males entering their 50s are likely to develop a malignancy in the prostate gland. The conventional treatment usually revolves around chemotherapy and radiation exposure, either preceding or following surgical removal of the prostate. The side effects – irregular bowel movements and difficulty in passing urine, male impotence and infertility and declining libido pave the way for depression and anxiety. But there is little cause for alarm because herbal life sciences offer very creative and life-sustaining solutions that if adopted can reduce a man's chances of succumbing to this disease and its side effects.

The basic symptoms that indicate prostate inflammation or enlargement

- Pain while passing urine

- Difficulty in emptying the bladder (feeling that something is obstructing passage)

- Frequent urination at night

- Delay in voiding urine

Useful and effective herbal remedies

Soybean products

Exceptionally high levels of DHT, a sex hormone, are known to provoke cancer malignancies in the prostate. The primary symptom is usually a localized inflammation that persists even after medication.   Regular weekly intake of soybean is very effective in suppressing cancer because soy contains agents that greatly inhibit DHT elevation. The only note of caution is to consume soy and soy products that are organically grown and processed, and which are non-GMO.

Vitamin D

Also known as the sunshine vitamin, it plays a proactive role in keeping the prostate healthy and active. Unfortunately, insufficient exposure to sun rays means the body doesn't get to replenish diminishing Vitamin D levels. Dairy products and seafood, if consumed in good quantities, ensure an abundant supply of the vitamin. But if your diet is low in dairy and seafood intake, the best way out is Vitamin D supplementation. Cholecalciferol (Vitamin D3) supplements in doses of 60,000 IU taken bi-monthly are very effective in combating prostate disorders. The vitamin also improves hormone balance and mood.

Lycopene

Another powerful lifesaver and prostate protector is Lycopene which is abundant in tomatoes, and in reasonably good quantity in watermelons and grapefruit. The best way is to puree tomato to a fine paste and to consume it liberally. It's even better if you add a dash of virgin olive oil and a couple of flakes of garlic to liven up the proceedings. Prepared this way, you have a potent prostate cancer buster ready to be consumed as a healthy sandwich. The results are powerful as the markers that indicate prostate cancer decline steadily as more lycopene steadily enters the system.

If you feel you are suffering some if not all of the classic symptoms indicating a malfunctioning prostate, your best approach should be a healthier diet followed up with regular outdoor activity, fresh air, and light exercise. Then, balance your lifestyle change with the herbal remedies we have suggested. The positive results should be forthcoming within a week of the treatment. If the symptoms persist (in 90 percent of cases, they won't), you're better off consulting a qualified health practitioner. If you are fortunate enough to consult a wise doctor, you'll be shown an integrated way of combining what modern medicine and herbal science can jointly deliver, causing minimum distress to your organs and health.

The men's guide to a healthier skin

It's not just women that are anxious about skincare – nowadays it's become priority number one for men too. Fortunately, you can stop reaching for over the counter ointments and salves that are loaded with skin destroying steroids and make do with herbal solutions that are risk-free and side effect free.

Combine two parts of the burdock and a portion of dandelion into a decoction. Once the roots are done simmering, introduce one portion of calendula and allow the decoction to steep for 10 to 15 minutes. After straining the cooled mixture, drink 3 to 4 cups daily, adding honey to create a delightful flavor.

Using the same ingredients and technique you can also prepare a strong infusion in larger batches which can be refrigerated for longer periods. You can use the infusion as a body wash just after your daily bath, allowing the infusion to dry out on the skin.

The strong antiviral, antibacterial properties of Calendula and Witch Hazel combine well for creating a potent skin cleanser and toner. The immediate task is to create a potent tincture using Calendula flowers soaked in Witch Hazel extract (Witch Hazel substituting for alcohol). Store the tincture in a capped bottle in the open and apply small portions to the acne affected skin using a cotton swab. You can leave the tincture to dry and there's no need to wash or rinse the skin after application. For refreshing facial skin, you can pour small quantities of the tincture into a hand sprayer, using it twice daily to preserve the youth and texture of shining skin.

Most adolescent skin types tend to be too oily and excessive use of oil-based skin creams may destroy the skin's suppleness and tone. The other extreme is the dry adolescent skin which if not properly moisturized could break out into rashes and pimples. For drier skin, it's best to combine white clay with a spoonful of jojoba, olive or grapeseed oil that can be applied twice a day to preserve good skin tone and healthy texture.

Needless to say, a diet that doesn't deliver sufficient quantities of Vitamin D and the B complex vitamins is a surefire recipe for unhealthy, lackluster skin. It's best to avoid foods that are rich in sugars and burnt carbon, especially foods that are commercially prepared containing ample quantities of rancid oils – all of which stress healthy skin. To preserve healthy skin, increase intake of dairy products and seafood, or resort to direct supplements, ensuring skincare in the long term.

The "fantastic four" herbal collection you can't ignore

Perhaps the best way of concluding this encyclopedia medicana is to list the kind of herbs that work major miracles in restoring health and improving vitality and virility. The last word (virility) should provoke more interest, especially in men. So, here we go!

1. **Herbs that promote health and wellbeing:** At the end of a hard day's night what a man craves for is a de-stressor, the kind that does not intoxicate but which rejuvenates the system, preparing the individual to become fighting fit for the following day. These are the herbs that not only do that bit also keep the hormones nicely balanced so that the day starts on an even keel and stays balanced throughout. The longer you use these herbs; the better will be your capacity to withstand the rigors of even the toughest work routine. The herbs that are up there in our pantheon of superheroes are ***Ashwagandha, Ginseng, Eleuthero, Rhodiola and Hawthorn*** which alone have the potential to bring out the best in you.

2. **Sour is simply sensational as far as the digestive system is concerned:** Bitters such as lemon, hops, dandelion, and artichoke give a powerful boost to liver function, aiding the liver in detoxifying the body slowly,

surely and systematically throughout the day. They also cool the body and maintain excellent pH balance, keeping acidity at bay. That's your window to freedom from a host of diseases that would otherwise overwhelm your digestive tract.

3. **Herbs that improve cardiac function and blood circulation:** The ancient healing arts are unanimous in projecting the heart to be the seat of our mental and emotional wellbeing. It is no wonder that severe depression and chronic anxiety often accompany cardiac distress and circulatory problems. Herbs like Valerian root, ginkgo, hawthorn, motherwort, and blueberry are uniquely equipped to revitalize the system and improve blood circulation. These powerful herbs help men overcome the blues and re-energize the spirit. A welcome side effect of long-term use of these herbs is increased libido and sexual chemistry that men will surely appreciate.

4. **Herbs that calm soothe and relax:** The restless mind, the fidgety nervous system, the exhaustion of intense hyperactivity, not to speak of sleep disturbances, all contribute to fatigue, depression, anxiety, and loss of sexual performance. The best herbal antidotes are Ashwagandha, chamomile, St. John's wort, lavender, kava and milky oats which go a long way in calming the neural synapses, balancing adrenaline levels and in restoring hormonal balance – the three essential requirements for a relaxed and calm body. The restorative and rejuvenating powers of these herbs are legendary. In short, these are the four herbal categories that ought to fill the power man's treasure chest of medicines.

Don't stop with our formulae and keep experimenting!

What we have documented is a broad and panoramic view of what herbal sciences offer for tackling a plethora of ailments and disorders that plague mankind. But the benefits are by no means confined to what we mention. Most of these herbs have such a great potential for healing that they may (unknown to you) heal even ailments that remain undetected by skilled physicians and sophisticated diagnostic tools.

The best of traditional herbal healing knowledge

To make the best use of herbs, study each herb individually. Trace the herb to its source of production. Talk to the people involved in the production and supply chain. Listen carefully to what they have to say regarding the herb's correct usage and potential. Handle, smell and observe the quality and texture of each herb so you get a clear idea of the quality and grading of the herb that you are eventually processing.

No herbalist can consider himself or herself to be the guru (or repository) of all knowledge, so it would be wise of you to read extensively and learn from what all the masters have to say regarding herbal healing power. This is the best way to gain a holistic perspective of this immensely rich source of healing power.

Please appreciate the pitfalls of online herbal research. Most blogs on herbs simply rehash content that is grossly outdated. Confine your research to sources that are well established, reputed and universally acknowledged for their credibility.

Your approach to herbal sciences should be as rational and objective as possible. Don't allow yourself to be taken in purely by the narrative that each treatise places before you. Experiment with each herb and assess its positive effects and analyze the side effects if any. If for any reason a herb does not seem to be producing the desired results or a herb may be causing more discomfort than healing, discard it and record a diary of its effects for future reference.

Herbs often work best in combinations and that's one of the chief reasons you'll find a lot of herbal remedies to be clusters of potent ingredients. You may rest assured that we have consciously avoided listing herbs that are controversial or which have gathered negative publicity. All the herbs listed here are safe and you can use them to your heart's content without having to bother about side effects. But, as we have cautioned earlier, you must avoid or discontinue herbs that are not suited to your system. In herbal sciences, it is universally accepted that what claims to work wonders for one persona need not hold true for another. The fault lies not in the efficacy or lack of potency in the herb but in our individual biochemistry that reacts differently to different herbs.

Take for instance Valerian root which is universally acknowledged to be a potent stabilizer of the nervous system producing a soothing effect in hyperactive and restless individuals and insomniacs. Though it is accepted to be safe, no toxic and non-addictive, the same herb can provoke an imbalanced response in some individuals. If you happen to be that rare specimen, you may observe that Valerian root makes you agitated and sleepless. If that's the case, you're better off discarding valerian in favor of something that may be better suited to you like Ashwagandha.

A word of caution as to where you source an herb. If something is coming to you neatly and attractively packaged and sold on the sly across a pharmaceutical counter, you're better off avoiding it altogether. Try sourcing herbs from farms and the producers directly as that gives you a golden opportunity to interact with a person that knows the product intimately. It's always safer to source an herb in its original form than having to deal with a processed product you have no idea about. It's difficult (sometimes impossible) to judge an herb's quality and stock once it is processed beyond recognition unless you're dealing with a reputed company. But why take the risk when you're investing in your health and wellbeing. So trudge that extra mile to the farm and ensure you're dealing in the genuine stuff. Most of these farms and community endeavors will be ethically compliant and wildcrafted to an herbalist's precise standards. Tonics, decoctions, and tinctures, if ordered online may leave you in doubt regarding the potency and efficacy of the mixture. You can set aside all doubts by taking total charge of the entire cycle from sourcing fresh herbs and processing to packaging (storing) the end product.

Never disregard or dismiss the debate on organic protocols versus artificially enhanced cropping practices.

That debate is not confined to scientists but affects you (the consumer) deeply. Most of what is expected from the healing energies within a herb works well only if the original product (the herb) is organically grown in a farm that is free of residual pesticides and artificial growth enhancers. Anything (any herb) that is even remotely connected to GMO practices is totally unsafe and is to be avoided at all costs.

Last but not the least, there's a huge community of herbal healers out there ready to help you sort out any starting nightmares if you feel yourself a complete novice in this dynamic field. As you interact more with knowledgeable people you will be inspired to start your own herbal farm even if you have limited access to land resources. Growing your own herbs is a fun way of adding value to your life. You may discover growing herbs to be the most creative adventure you've ever attempted. Happy hunting and healthy healing to you and your entire family!

One last thing!

I want to give you a **one-in-two-hundred chance** to win a **$200.00 Amazon Gift card** as a thank-you for reading this book.

All I ask is that you give me some feedback, so I can improve this or my next book :)

Your opinion is *super valuable* to me. It will only take a minute of your time to let me know what you like and what you didn't like about this book. The hardest part is deciding how to spend the two hundred dollars! Just follow this link.

http://reviewers.win/herbalmen